SLOWING DOWN FOR SANITY
A LOSER'S SURVIVAL GUIDE
(*FUNNY OR SERIOUS? YOU'LL JUST HAVE TO READ-ON AND SEE FOR YOURSELF!)

ROBERT L. BOYER*
(* WELL-QUALIFIED LOSER)

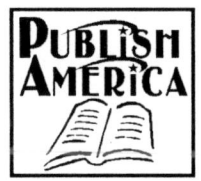

PublishAmerica
Baltimore

© 2002 by Robert L. Boyer.
All rights reserved. No part of this book may be reproduced in any form without written permission from the publishers, except by a reviewer who may quote brief passages in a review to be printed in a newspaper or magazine.

First printing

ISBN: 1-59286-498-8
PUBLISHED BY PUBLISHAMERICA BOOK
PUBLISHERS
www.publishamerica.com
Baltimore

Printed in the United States of America

Acknowledgements

How does it go, again? "Behind every great man stands..."

Well, I'm not so great, and no one is really standing behind me or shoring-me-up. I'm just addicted to cliches, which by reading further, you'll soon tire of. Just can't stop.

To business:

Writing this rambling wreck of a book has been a stealthy enterprise. Largely stealing time from work before the day began, or long after the last phone calls came in. (Except for some scribbling by the pool or at the bookstore café.)

The most difficult thing was maintaining a consistent tone and/or mood. Writing in installment fashion is far more trying than seclusion for weeks on end. It requires re-immersing yourself in the rhythm and style at each sitting—regardless of outside events or emotional state. That I've salvaged any sense of cogency is perhaps my greatest accomplishment.

Hitting appropriate topics wasn't any easier. I tried—in semi-scientific fashion—to pick them based on a combination of personal experience, universality, and humor. Humor will keep them reading, but without that ole ring-of-truth, there's no real point to it. I've used this formula with success on some topics, less successfully on others. You be the judge and jury here.

I started writing as an outgrowth of my still-ongoing therapy. First, for myself (supposedly very good for one's mental health). But why not share? (Maybe even make a few dollars at the same time). So here we are.

Now, to people:

Thanks to Kathy, my therapist, for encouraging me to write down my thoughts and experiences. She's right—it does help.
Kudos to Dave Barry and Billy Crystal—my inspirations.
Thanks to Roger Bernstein and Linda Osberg-Braun, my 'bosses,' for putting up with all this s__t. Anyway, they gave me a job when I needed one. 'Nough said.
A sincere thank you to Sydney Marks and Maria Elena Buria, for reasons best known to them. Two of the finest individuals I have been privileged to know in my life.
To my Ex, Maxine, for her sense of humor as well as common sense. And for continuing to be a friend. 20-plus years of shared experiences are a big slice-of-life. Thanks, Max.
Thanks to Mom and Dad—which words are woefully inadequate to express. In particular, for reading excerpts over breakfast and critiquing. In general, for always being there.
My kids, Jackie and Richard. They're what life is all about. I dedicate this book to them.

Aventura, Florida   February 27, 2002

SLOWING DOWN FOR SANITY

Have you ever experienced any of the following:

You get up at 6:15 am, trying to get a head start on the day. Rush to shave, shower, down an orange juice and vitamin, and rush to the car. You get on the road, and whoa:
Everyone else is out there, and the grand prix has started in earnest.

Drivers are darting about, like Daytona 500 maniacs trying to get 1-2 car lengths ahead. As if this will make their day. People cut you off left and right, and the police are there too, trying to write as many tickets as possible.

You get to work—early. However, once the calls and business begin, it's like you're a tortoise from another dimension. Everyone else is moving in fast forward. As if to stop and breathe will make the whole house of cards come crashing down. Bosses and supervisors hover over you—asking about this and that and barking orders. You attack one work project—but the boss says drop that 5 minutes later, and do this. The scenario repeats itself all morning.

Comes noon, and you escape on your walk. Perhaps to have lunch—that is, if your stomach can handle it. When you return, if it's been more than 25 minutes, the dirty looks catch you.

You're also told that an emergency has arisen, and that it's all (or mostly) your fault. You conclude that to leave the premises even for that brief respite is to invite danger, and threaten job security.

The afternoon lurches on in top gear—repeating the morning pace and anxieties.

Comes 5 p.m., and NO ONE leaves. Comes 5:30, and still no progress towards the door. Maybe by 6. At least 6, if not 6:30. Then it seems safe to depart without risking demerits.

Back into the grand prix—seems to go on through the evening. You arrive home totally wasted—mentally, emotionally, and physically, as the cumulative result of—dare I use the word—STRESS!

Seem familiar? We all feel this nonsense. But we've been trained to remain silent. Why?

Because mentioning it makes you a loser, a malcontent, a slouch. Even un-American!!

We're programmed to buy into the notion that ours is an age of unprecedented prosperity. That work is more rewarding than ever; and that we have an exceptional 'quality of life.' What bullshit.

Yes, salaries are higher than ever. Otherwise, life is worse in every quantitative dimension. Twenty or so years ago, the workday ran from 9-5. Eight hours. Now it runs from 7:30 to 6; or 7; or 8. And that's expected—not rewarded. And that's not counting the commute. Twenty years ago, we got in the car at 8. If we did that now, we'd never arrive at work. You've got to get on the road before 7. The drive home takes another hour.

Twenty years ago an employee's lunch hour was his/her time—sacred. Now it's simply tolerated as a necessary fuel stop.

Twenty years ago there was some civility in relations between employees and between employer - employee. Today, it's who can beat down the other best. Survival of the meanest.

We don't do or say anything—we can't 'risk' our jobs. We keep these observations deep inside, obscured from public view. Ashamed of our weakness. Feeling we're the only one.

Wake up!! Let's be honest—we ALL feel this. We're ruining our lives in the quest for—nothing. It's time to stop and smell the roses before they disappear.

In this book, I'm advocating the birth of a revolution: slowing down for sanity. The corporate world will fight tooth and nail, and use every known scam to dissuade us. But the truth is—we have the power to make our lives slower, simpler, more humane, more balanced. We can start today—each person on their own, one at a time, until it becomes apparent that a kinder gentler life is resurfacing. Like a long-lost friend. This is exciting stuff—and I now ask you to join me in this journey.

What a mistake to live for vacations

Everyone loves a vacation. Just the word makes your mouth water with anticipation. We pour through the travel section looking for great deals and basking in the visual images. The thought itself provides a warm glow.

Did you ever wonder why we dream about a 1-week vacation months in advance? Hey, stupid—it's because our daily lives are so miserable and fraught with tension. The vacation promises relief from traffic, schedules, deadlines, pressure, you name it. We conveniently avoid reading the 'fine print'; i.e., that it only lasts a week.

Inevitably, vacations are a disaster. I hate to make you re-live this scenario, but lets go through it, anyway:

First, there's the "getting ready" part. I'm not just talking about wardrobe shopping and packing. I'm referring to the 'tying—up-the-loose-ends' at work, before the grand escape.

You try to put out all the fires before you leave—you actually think it can be accomplished. You can't do it. Today's pressurized workplace is merely a constant continuum of emergencies. So, at 3 p.m. on your last day before the big V, a crisis pops up. It can't be solved—so you delegate resolution to a not-so-happy subordinate or co-worker. OK—you leave with 2-3 crises and (if we're honest, here) 4-5 deadlines which will come up during the ensuing week while you're ensconced in Maui.

Then something strange happens: it takes you 2 full days to slow down and let worklife turn from a searing flame into a fuzzy glow. Finally, 3 days in, you get into the groove. Fine for 3 days. Then, as sure as death and taxes, you start stressing a full 2 days before the return.

The feeling returning to your office the day after vacation is akin to cardiac symptoms: cold sweat; cramped neck; sour stomach. All in anticipation of walking back onto the minefield. This isn't paranoia—what you fear (the crises out of control; the deadlines somehow missed; the attitudes from staff) all comes true. If you haven't had your immediate heart attack, almost certainly you will end that first day saying under your breath: "I need a vacation."

In summary, vacations solve nothing - they don't relieve anxiety; they enhance it. Vacations are an impotent panacea for coping. What you really have to do is change your daily life. More vacation time only makes the stark contrast worse.

So, take that time—that trip you've been scouting-out. But see it for what it is - merely a getaway, not Zanax.

Watch-out for the 'Thirtysomethings'

Meanwhile, back at the ranch, you try desperately to get up-to-speed. I mean, every last ounce of strength to have that 'edge' again.

But you can't get on the bosses's good side. He/she's out to squeeze that last ounce of energy from you, for that whim-of-the-moment urgent project.

Be ready to be pounded, hounded, scorned, joked-at, and otherwise ignored.

You see—what you've got here is a 'Thirtysomething.' Say what?

A '30-something' can't be entirely defined or described. Let me try my best:

This creature appears in human form, male or female, commonly between the ages of 25-35. By this time, they've usually risen to mid-level supervisory positions—taking special pride in being 'fast-tracked.' They wear the latest trends in clothing, and rarely dress casually.

'30-S's' are incredibly self-centered. It defines them. Their entire being is focused upon getting ahead and reaching the next plateau in their career. Understandable—career is everything to them; even family comes second. Sure, they will act and say what is politically correct: contributions to the right charities; driving cars/SUVs in current vogue; supporting currently-popular causes and candidates; eating the 'right' foods.

Make no mistake about it: these affectations are for appearances, only. Appearances are what counts in their insatiable drive to the top. The 30-S has no real core beliefs. (Shallow is a mild word to describe him/her). A true Machiavellian, the 30-S will use you, your co-worker, sex, chicanery, whatever, to maneuver around seeking advantage. You best watch-out.

Most of us 'oldsters' cope with the 30-S by taking the easy path of least resistance. Rather than upset the 30-S and risk being attacked, we grin and bear it. We follow directions; drop one project and delve into the newly-assigned task (as disjointed an approach as that may be); offer apologies for matters entirely outside of our control. Anything to placate the 30-S and hopefully take their focus away from us.

This approach is rarely successful. The 30-S learns that we are a passive prey, easily dominated. They will return for the kill time after time.

The venerable Vince Lombardi supposedly said: "The best defense is an offense." Correct, sir. Listen to the ranting, but talk back. Consider the proposals or stream-of-consciousness task abruptly assigned, and critique the idea. Work hard and complete your projects. But don't stay till 9 p.m. just to impress your boss. Talk REAL to the 30-S. I guarantee that the 30-S will eventually shut-up.

The 30-S, when so approached, will listen—because it has no self-confidence. With all their apparent bravado, the 30-Somethings have that Achilles heel. I'm not sure why, but it certainly explains much of their obnoxious behavior.

The 30-S is deathly afraid that the world will discover this weakness. Play on it; and you will put the 30-S in his/her place.

The more aggressive you are in defending your rights and position, the less likely being hounded. Try it.

(Sigh) Well…eventually the 30-Something will suffer some hard knocks in life and mature to a degree. Like us. I wish them only the best. (Isn't that the politically correct thing to say?)

If only I had money, I'd…

…open a coffee shop in Colorado or dish out ice cream all day long. Ah yes, the fantasy!! The ultimate escape!! The simpler life; the small store on the corner; even retirement. Conventional wisdom says you'll get bored. You won't. If done right, the world will slow down around you and come alive. Alive in the very vivid sense of conversations that linger; smells and tastes that can be savored; pride in a small job well done; music and art that envelops, not merely serving the purpose of soothing raw nerves. Yes, my dear friends—the symphony of life!!

A cornucopia of self-help books address this subject, preying on our shared desire to escape the rat race, and offering approaches which allow the dream on a shoestring. Fagetaboutit!!

If you want it, go for it—but you need the bucks. Don't kid yourself. Otherwise, Einstein, you'll be trading one set of stresses for another. That's no way to smell the roses!

So no financing. No long-term contracts and franchise fees. No partners (partnerships fail at a predictably higher rate than marriages). My Mom says: "Live within your means." She's right (bless her). Make the 'Great Escape' after you make the money.

Where does it come from? Trees? Right! Sorry, Charlie, you can't make it happen. It will rain money if and when the Big Guy chooses. Should lightening strike, go for it! Don't waste a minute; otherwise the mundane will surely encroach and hold you back.

If the bolt hits, don't:
1. Buy the Porsche.
2. Get the Big House on the Beach.
3. Stay on the job for more than 30 days (you should give notice, you know).

Do:
1. Stay on the job for up to 30 days.
2. Put new tires on the car.
3. Say your goodbyes, and go!

I know…you're disappointed. This schmuck is telling you to change your life, but not telling you how. Listen—I'm saying if it happens; if you awake one morning flush, buy the coffee shop. No-brainer, Bub.

By the way, I almost forgot, you can improve the odds by pursuing the following:

Stay close with rich relatives; and buy Lotto tickets (hey, at least meet God half-way).

And While You're at it, Get Some Exercise

Sometimes conventional wisdom is right. Regular exercise DOES help. I see that more when I fall off the wagon than when I'm humming along.

But you've got to go at it like you brush your teeth and take a shower. Every day; and don't even think about it. It has to be routine.

Here's the short list of cardiovascular, calisthenic, and upper body workout venues:

A. You can join a health club; or resort to the poorman's:

B. Home-grown hodgepodge.

Take the health clubs (please). They're not for everyone. First, they cost money (the last thing you need is another monthly payment). Second, you have to drive there. Third, they provide too many distractions to enjoy a major benefit of working-out: time to think.

I prefer the home-grown variety. This is a good one (coincidentally, it's mine):

A. Pushups. Several sets in the morning; and again at night before turning in. Every other day.

B. Torso and knee bends (same schedule).

C. Brisk walks (not jogs or runs).
D. Swimming laps (in season or when available).

After a month, you'll see results.
Don't stop. Once you lose momentum, you're finished. Again, make it a Pavlovian routine—like bathing.
What will it do for you?
1. You'll feel better.
2. You'll lose some weight and inches.
3. You'll have time to think—in peace.

Believe me, it's the latter benefit that you'll appreciate most. Particularly on those brisk a.m. or p.m. walks. You can think through relationships, work issues, etc. Mostly-interpersonal relationships.

Walks provide time to replay events and conversations verbatim. No phones or beepers to interrupt; i.e., no distractions (other than the occasional greeting to a fellow ambulator). You'll also notice that the world around you is slowing down. Your senses will come alive with the smells of foliage, food, and—unfortunately—diesel trucks. In return, I guarantee a sense of renewal and well-being. Start your weekend this way, and set the tone for a marvelous time on a different dimensional wavelength.

Try it and see. Just one proviso, please: no Walkman. Come on, you can do without it for an hour!

Stay Sexual—Stay Young

If you told me that your sex drive's gone down the shitter, it wouldn't surprise me. Been there—done that. Might as well have no sexual organs at all. They seem to serve no purpose. Dead weight.

YOU ARE NOT ALONE! If we held a convention of sexual corpses, we'd fill Yankee Stadium to the brim. Seems like the faster our society goes, the less we copulate, etc.

This is not in our minds—it's for real. The correlation exists.

As we bemoan the loss of sexual appetite, let's take stock of the residual fallout:

Permeating everything is the absence of intimacy. No longer do we share inner thoughts and bare our souls to each other. Competitiveness is enhanced. Empathy a dim memory. We focus on the lust for material things—the prestigious car, the bigger house. As if this lust is the misdirected replacement for human relationships.

Do you doubt? OK. How many times, recently, have you had an entire evening of warmth, intimacy, soul-baring conversation, interspersed with tender sex? You know, the kind of night where the TV is off, time floats ethereally, and the sounds of the trees and our own voices weave a wistful duet? (Don't I write well!)

I think I've had maybe 2 of those nights in my entire life. That's it. And you know what? That interpersonal 'melding' helped to briefly put life in better perspective. Fleeting as that was, it tells me something. That our everyday value system is fucked-up, and that lack of intimacy and physical bonding contribute to these twisted values. Clearly.

There's a risk in sexual bonding and intimacy. If you really open up, the imperfections and dirty laundry will show. We've been programmed to fear that. (Remember the Thirtysomethings?) But you've got to cross that bridge (I keep telling myself the same thing). Baring and sharing the bad things strengthens closeness. And it makes for better sex.

Try it. If I'm wrong, you'll become a monk and throw my book away. But if I'm right, you owe me lunch. I hope to have free meals for the rest of my life!

Honesty and the Truth

I'm going to be deadly serious for a bit. (Just a bit, I promise.) We probably expend 50% of our daily energies in obscuring the truth. Dishonesty, evasion, spin-doctoring—whatever you call it—is a major stressor. We lie all day long, to the point that we don't even consciously recognize this counterproductive activity anymore.

Why? Because we fear confrontation.

We want to go about our lives in a Pleasantville, even Disneyesque fashion, where everyone smiles and there are no hard choices. Fifty years of sitcoms, from *Father Knows Best* to the *Sopranos*, encourage this fear of confrontation. (Betty vs. her Father; Tony and his shrink). It's the embrace of the predictable, and the aversion to surprise.

"People should like me." Accepting this maxim, we adapt every conversation, indeed every interaction, to achieve this aura of agreeability. A state of bliss with no apparent storms brewing.

What a crock. Holding off the storm clouds, real or imagined, only breeds tornados. I should know. Happens to me all the time. (My stop and start therapy deals consistently with this issue.) Lying is intoxicating: things go along well for awhile, then the shit hits the fan. Whatever negative would have resulted from an originally truthful statement is compounded exponentially by the ensuing coverup. It goes without saying that one is much better-off being truthful from the get-go. You and I understand this intellectually, then go off merrily and deceive anyway.

We pay a high price for this. Emotionally. And stress-wise. You've got to know that once you weave the web of lies, you can't stop. You've got to maintain it. On top of all your other chores and projects, you need to constantly plot your next line in advance. The spin gets faster and faster, till you're swamped in it—and it explodes out of control.

If anything makes life become a whirling dervish, this is it.

Whew—I need to slow down. Just putting this into words is unnerving. And scary.

As we know by now, life is racing along fast enough. The last thing we need is trying to falsely tame it while fueling the lunacy at the same time.

Break the habit. Go cold-turkey. Try the truth and see if I'm right. Seriously, this might be the single, biggest step towards changing your life.

(Hey—and drop the co-payment in the box on your way out!)

Eating Large—Go For It!

My girlfriend and I LOVE chocolate cake. Oh, not just any chocolate cake. It's got to be just so—deep layers of fudge, smothered in dark chocolate chips, and topped with real whipped cream. Vanilla ice cream on the side, and (of course) two forks!!

It's become a weekend ritual (followed by pangs of guilt and days of fasting).

I've got to watch it, or I'll blossom. God Bless her, she won't gain nary an inch or pound.

We look forward to our frenzy as if it were a religious experience. Really, it gives us such joy! What the hell is going on here?

My friends, we are participating in an age-old American tradition: Eating Large.

Yes, it's boom and bust-out-all-over in our neck of the woods. And you know, that's OK, once or twice a week. Why not? Good food—rich food—fills the senses. You have a good time, and a wonderful shared experience. A very personal experience, and one which negates the need for big cars, fancy jewelry, and climbing the social strata.

You can't do it every night. Not only would it lose it's attractive qualities, but you'd blow your budget and wreak havoc physically. As they say, all good things in moderation.

But do it. It will fill your life in many ways: providing topics for conversation, and wistful memories waiting to be revisited. It will lend itself towards savoring the moment, while the rest of the world continues flying by. Good riddance.

Here's my "A" list of foods for joy:
1. Chocolate cake.
2. 'Real' wonton soup.
3. Marinated churrasco steak.
4. Homemade mashed potatoes with equally-impressive gravy.
5. A VERY dry, red wine.
6. Snickers bars.

The rest of the week you can eat this:
1. All-Bran.
2. Cranberry juice.
3. Grapefruit.
4. Garden salad.
5. Boiled chicken.

Look, there's no 'free lunch.' You indulge, you diet. Indulge, diet. (Nice rhythm, don't you think?) Wax on, wax off. Same thing. The yin and yang of life. Balance.

Isn't that amazing? I ended this section on a philosophical note!

Therapists

Today's my regular weekly appointment with Kathy. (No, she's my therapist)

I've been going to Kathy off and on for almost a year. The last stint is now entering its 4th month. Counseling is a good thing. It'll slow you down, and create a manageable framework for daily living.

With one proviso: finding the right therapist. Which is (here we go with the cliches, again) a needle in a haystack.

There seem to be 3 types:

A. Passive bordering on inert.
B. The Generalist.
C. Opinionated (but finds you boring).

Incidentally (as if you couldn't guess), I've had one of each. Here's the rundown:

Carlos is a nice enough guy. That is, if you can judge him by his note-taking and smiling grunts alone. That's all he would do: take notes and grunt. This got me nowhere. I mean, I talk to myself all the time anyway. I don't need to pay for the experience.

Karen loves the obvious. She expounds on the world's general state of affairs, and how we have to cope with it. She'll ask: "How do you manage with all your responsibilities?" Answer: "I don't know. It gives me a lot of stress." Response: "You see!! It's not you; the world is very stressful, today." That would be followed, in short order, by: "You see!! Relationships are complicated; You see!! Life is too short"; "You see!! The moon is not made of cheese." I went to Karen twice.

Kathy (my current) takes a pro-active role. She presses me on the issues. She starts each session wanting a progress report on the past week. This I like. The sessions fly by. Usually, I've shot my load in the first 30 minutes. I know—from a surreptitious glance at my watch.

Kathy gives advice, but I think she's bored at times. I find her looking away (when she thinks I'm not watching). It makes me feel I'm a bit trite and not all that interesting. In any event, that might be all in my head.

I get books to read. Since I probably have some sort of adult A.D.D., I generally flit from section to section, catching what I can. Having a book on hand is a valuable prop for the ensuing week. My girlfriend and parents steal it and provide impromptu reviews. At best, it reinforces the topic at hand. At worst, just a shrug or a yawn. Depends on the writer—not the subject material. On balance, though, the reading reinforces the advice. That's the advantage to an assertive therapist. There are lessons to learn—and interceding speeds the process along until that proverbial bell goes off in your head which says: "Gee—that has the ring of truth".

I'll continue with Kathy until my insurance runs out. It just feels good. Having a pro-active therapist gives you that slower, calming feeling when you walk out. It makes you verbalize—that's good.

We all need to talk to someone. You might go through a dozen psychs/MSWs/whatevers before settling down for the long haul. If you're in that rut, don't give up. You'll know the right one when you get there. You WILL get there. And it's worth the ride!

Living with Parents

I've been living with my folks for the last 9 months. It's very cozy: their Florida condo has 2 bedrooms, and I've got the front one. Well, actually, I think it's a closet converted into a bedroom. That's about the size of it. The 'bed' is a fold-out loveseat. After nine months, the springs are announcing their presence. I shouldn't complain—it's rent free.

Have you ever wondered what its like to regress from 49 to 14? Live with your folks. You'll stay young—you have no choice! You have to report on your comings-and-goings, what you ate and will eat, how late you're staying out, and if you spoke with anyone in the past 8 hours. And become a good listener. That's a prerequisite.

Now I'm going to tell you something invaluable. Living with your parents is one of the best gifts you can give yourself—at least during transitions.

If you're like me, you've moved in out of necessity. Typically a marital/relationship break-up, financial crisis, or—most likely—a combination of both. Before you moan over this turn of events, tell yourself: God bless ! This could be one of the most rewarding events of adult mid-life. For you—and for them.

The opportunity to experience renewed closeness with parents at this stage in life is priceless. Your mother and father are perhaps (aside from the kids) the only people on the planet who show you unconditional love. This is both a comfort and a lesson. Realizing that is calming in the truest sense. Bask in it, but participate.

By this time, hopefully, you realize that age = experience = a keen understanding of human nature. Particularly frailty and weakness. If you're honest and open, they won't be judgmental. Isn't that refreshing? And their insights are right on target.

It took me awhile. But I can truly say that I now share 'life' with my folks more than ever before, and that I value their opinion and love. It's so rewarding. And it's there for the asking.

I'll move into my own place soon (that is, as soon as I get a modification in my child support). But I hope that the lessons I've learned from this period together will linger.

Truly, life unfolds in mysterious ways. Something is taken from you, and you get something marvelous in return.

Mom and Dad—if you're reading this, Thanks!! I love you lots.

Ex's

Ex-spouses; ex-girlfriends; ex-boyfriends. Ex's. They permeate our lives. Ever-present reminders of failures and good memories. Both. And prime shapers of future behavior.

We can't pass a day without their intrusions. From child-support payments to wistful thoughts of 'what could have been', the presence of our former partners lingers far longer than the relationship itself.

This can drive you crazy, adding stress upon stress. Or you can approach the issue constructively. That's the key to Ex-management. (I'm looking for that key right now!)

There are several basic Rules to successfully dealing with the Ex-Factor:

1. No head games.
2. Pay your child support.
3. Socialize with the opposite gender.
4. Expand your circle of friends.
5. Have a life plan.
6. Write a book.

As if you couldn't guess, we'll discuss them one-by-one.

Do not; repeat, do not play head games with your ex. What's a 'head game'? Simply speaking, that's where we create a false scenario devised (solely) to get a rise out of the other. Here's a basic and common one: avoiding contact to appear uninterested. Get a life—you're interested. You just want to make your other cry 'Uncle' first. You want to show that your Ex is no longer of any daily concern to you.

And the result? The fixation on the head game perpetuates the Ex's presence and control over your life. Just the opposite of the impression you're trying to make. Every morning you count the days you've avoided contact as if it were a trophy. The truth is, your Ex couldn't care less. Meanwhile, your daily game eats you up alive.

Get a life! Be natural, and let the relationship slowly die at its own pace. Don't go for the cheap thrill of gaining satisfaction, revenge, whatever. That only keeps the flame of the relationship burning. You don't want that. (Or do you?)

Now, to THE paramount rule of all: Make your support payments. Timely. Pay your Ex before you even buy lunch. I can't emphasize this enough. If you falter, the Wrath of God will come crashing down from the heavens. It will literally destroy your life.

If you've read this far, it's fair to assume you suffer from acute stress. Imagine adding this to your plate: hourly calls from the Ex; abuse from the kids; being dragged into court; facing a cynical judge; going to jail. And that's not even counting the arrears. If you're living from check-to-check (like me), you'll never pay off the arrears.

Unless you have a death wish, be smart—pay on time. Even better—pay ahead. I'll tell you—if I got a windfall, I'd calculate the total support remaining and pay it lump sum now. Alacazam!! No more Ex; one less stress!! (That's cute)

With this neutralized, readjust your focus to socializing. With the opposite sex. There's a whole other world out there, Mac.

Go out and get it. Have some fun!

You can go to the local jazz bar and drink. You can get fixed-up. You can go to singles events. You can rush into another relationship. Advice from school of hard-knocks: chuck the latter, and enjoy the first three.

The LAST thing you need is another relationship. Maybe never; certainly not now. First of all, you're not financially ready. Secondly, if you're like me, you need the experience of living solo. You have no sense of self. Simple things are foreign to you: like making your own meals, cleaning the house (apartment), making dinner, setting a schedule, balancing your checkbook. We're talking about getting to know yourself. Caring for your own needs. Rush into a relationship, and you miss this opportunity. It happened to me.

Have some fun!! Dating starts awkwardly. You need a roadmap. It's a learn-as-you-go exercise, but it gets easier. Really, it does. Here're two places to start: a business meeting or card exchange; an organized singles event. Try the business venue first.

Oh—bring some cards with you. (You don't want to be fishing for a pen later). Dress nice. And talk a blue streak. About anything and everything—other than meeting someone. That's right, keep it light—but impersonal. Collect enough cards and you can follow-up with any number of people. You think you're the only one there with a hidden agenda? They're all looking to meet someone—indirectly. Try it out and see for yourself. By the way, these events are usually CHEAP. Sometimes totally free!!

Mix the business networking with singles dances, cocktail hours, whatevers. Approach these with the lowest of expectations. This will reduce your anxiety. I'll tell you what works for me: people-watching. It's the greatest. Short, tall, slinky, low-cut, big hair, no hair, you'll see it all. Grab a seat at the bar—and watch. See the maneuvers and eye-contact. See who's with whom. Observe body language. What a show! You can observe with passive fascination—or, if you're ready, you can participate.

Just be natural and smile. After all, you're happy to be there. And drink in moderation. You don't need a ticket (or worse) on the way home.

You might make a friend. Which brings me to that subject. (Notice the segue) Wake up, fool. Everyone needs friends; probably now more than ever. If you have one, you're lucky. You might only have acquaintances from work. That doesn't count. A real Pal is a gift. Someone you can share with: movies; dinners; sports; thoughts. All without sexual tension or other related expectations.

A friend refocuses your life. More than one enriches it. They're hard to find and harder to keep. The key is: choose carefully.

You can't be taught how to choose carefully. It's a trial-by-error process (like too much of life). Just keep your eyes open for the right qualities. Optimally (nice word), you want a friend who's better than you. Not richer, just better qualities: more honest; more trustworthy; more tolerant; more funny. Someone you can look up to and someone who can inspire the best in you. To make you 'stretch' a bit.

You'll know you've got a friend when you can show all your dirty laundry without flinching. And share without keeping score. Enjoy true friendship, and your focus on the Ex will fade into black. Wouldn't that be wonderful?

OK. So now that you've refocused and ex-orcised the Ex, where do we go from here?

I don't know about you, but I've always had to organize.

Write down to-do lists every day. (I never accomplish what I set out to do, but it makes me feel better). I think it has something to do with controlling one's life. Making lists seems to work, at least a bit. So—how about making the BIGGEST list of all?

A 'Life Plan.' Really, it's just a bigger version of your daily senility list. Covering the next 24 or so years instead of 24 hours. On every subject and concern imaginable.

This is your life—if you're going to plan it, make it go where you want. Don't be realistic—go for it! Big dreams. Doing what you've always wanted to do.

Close your eyes and clear out the gunk. Picture yourself at work or play. What's in the picture? Bingo! That's your life plan. Write it down. (Illustrate it if you want.)

Now—how does it feel? Come on, don't you feel better? Just having the thoughts and ideas are a boost. You may never get to the Promised Land, but the anticipation is at least half a thrill. You feel like you're on a road going someplace, and not just (getting biblical again) wandering in the desert.

Want to take the list/life plan exercise a step further? Write a book. Any book (well, other than a historical biography). Use a pad, pen, or computer. Put down your thoughts as they surface (that's what I'm doing right now). Don't follow an enforced outline, and you'll be surprised by the results.

Immediately, a palpable sense of calm will enfold you. A better sense of self. And control. I don't know for sure why this works. It just does. Continue on a daily basis. This will extend the sense of serenity. I think it's like painting or composing—creating something that's indelibly yours. And that's aside from your sense of accomplishment.

So what does this all have to do with Exs? Nothing, directly. But if you're occupied, if your focus changes, the emotional energies are spent elsewhere. That's the trick, friend.

You can't put the Ex behind if you don't have a life.
   Go out and get it!!

Holidays Without Stress (an extinct species)

Merry Christmas (Ho-Ho-Ho!!) Happy Chanukah! Happy Thanksgiving!

I just got through the Thanksgiving weekend. Put it this way—I survived it.

Let me tell you, these 'Holiday' weekends are human rollercoasters. There are enough ups, downs, and sideway turns to disable the most iron of stomachs. Who to visit; what (and how much) to eat; sending cards bulk-rate. Not to mention presents. I need *two* days of counseling this week—not just the usual session.

'Survival' IS the word. We need a guidebook to arrive at the finish line unscathed. Stress has to be the name of the mythological God of Holidays. If the food doesn't kill you, stress will. There's only one way to get by: invite everyone to your place. (And I do mean everyone). Here's how:

Start early. Very early. You're going to get invitations a month in advance, so send your invites two months out. That seems safe.

To avoid the usual recriminations, call (or e-mail) everyone you can think of. That includes Mom, Dad, Uncle Funny, your kids, your squeeze, your boss, your Ex, and your Ex's friends (who used to be your friends). Don't leave anyone out who could, conceivably, invite you. Now you're safe. More work, but less stress.

Don't panic—most won't be coming. Get ready for every excuse in the book and then some: "I'm going to my Mom's"; "We're going away"; "Tony's a vegan"; "No offense, but I don't like you." But you've solved your problem—no time-splitting schedule, and a generous reputation to boot. Those that actually show really want to be with you.

Then there's the eating. (I'm bloating-up just by the thought). Oi vay!! There's no solution to this dilemma. Coat your stomach in advance, and dig-in. Grab the appetizers; have some turkey; pass the brisket, please?; those yams look good; make room for dessert; down a cognac. Always remember to be sociable, and sing out loud: "I've had too much; fa-la-la-la-la, la-la, la-la". Recovery requires a 10-mile walk.

Finally, you need to deal with presents. Cut your losses and exercise some damage control. Get wine for adults; money for the kids. Wine is classy, and no one has any clue what it cost. The kids don't like clothes or books—but will happily take your cash.

Figure out the budget now. Otherwise, you're in big trouble.

Yes, Holidays are a wonderful time. The warmth of family and close friends. The joy of giving. The greetings of strangers. (I'm dripping in sentimentality.) If you approach them right, you'll make it through. I've got to remind myself of this: Christmas, Hanukah, and New Year's are coming. Better get the invitations out now!!

My Life as a Car

A bit of conventional wisdom: Boys become men, but they don't give up toys. The toys just become bigger. And more expensive.

This is true. Particularly with cars. Important to all men, some actually live and breathe them. The size, the speed, paint, leather, audio, wheels…and engines. Got to have power, and more of it!

When we're not driving, we're buying. And when we're not buying, we're tinkering. Tinker, tinker, tinker—till we drive the women totally crazy. They just can't understand us. Sorry, girls, it must be the male brain/female brain thing. Just live with it.

Cars are like an alternate reality. Immerse yourself, and you're transported to another planet. (Beam me up, Scotty!) I think it has something to do with immediate gratification. Seeing results for your hands-on efforts. Get a used example of what you've always wanted, and you'll know what I mean.

The challenge is in the fixin'. Making it better than it was this morning. Make it shine; make it fly. Get out the tools, wax, and rags. Start those wrenches!

Nothing (not even great sex) can match the satisfaction of a better ride through your own sweat and scrapes. It's like being melded together—the car and you. It lives! You live! The curmudgeon asks: How can one invest such emotional energy in a bucket of bolts? The mere asking of the question betrays a pitiful lack of understanding. Don't trust anyone like this. They're like people who hate dogs. Cold and calculating. Not like you—full of zest with grandiose delusions.

And you're not crazy. Neither are you alone in this mania. All you need to do is check out the magazine rack at the market. Compare the number of auto mags to news weeklies. No contest! Also note the prominent display of nearly-nude girls on the covers, alongside Impalas and 911's. Yes, sir. Cars are sexual. No doubt about it.

Important, too. Not just for transportation. For the void they fill. As well as the erasure of the past week's travails. Nothing— and I mean nothing—can replace the feeling of cruising in your car when it's on top of its game. Talk about stress reduction, this is it!

Personally, I'm partial to used Mercedes. Mercedes don't grow old—they age like fine wine. In particular, they crave TLC. Fix a part once, and it'll last forever. Polish the wood, and the fine grain will virtually emanate warmth. Nothing screams like quality. Restore the Benz to its former self, and you restore yourself. It's intoxicating. Must be others like me out there. You can get a 40-year-old part at the local dealer as easy as a fan belt on a Chevy. How sweet it is—but I digress.

Right now, my silver bullet is smiling. Just got its exotic shock absorbers re-tuned. When it's happy, I'm happy. But like a vacationer on a binge, it always wants more. So I'm making a list. And checking it twice. (What's with these Christmas tunes that run through my head?)

Go out and get your bullet. Find one that says: "I want a home," and adopt it. Buy low and pay cash. No payments—

just elbow grease and parts.

Treat it like a Lady, and Saturday mornings with tools-in-hand will make your world a better place. Just wait till your Saturday nights behind the wheel!

Brothers and Sisters

In a perfect world, our siblings would be our best friends. They would ooze the same unconditional love that we share with our parents.

You know differently. Brothers and sisters SOMETIMES get along—but, more often than not, it's a perfunctory relationship. A call or two every other month, and a visit over (dare I say) the Holidays. A relationship of appearances and obligation. But nothing much beneath the surface.

How sad. This is not a humorous topic. It's serious stuff. And it's not isolated—it's rampant. Just that it doesn't seem that way. People and families keep up appearances—so you don't know who else suffers from dysfunctional family syndrome. Once again, if it's any solace, know that the majority of family units are like yours. We're just too ashamed to admit it.

Here's why: like it or not, we live in the land of "should do." Individually and societally, Americans uniformly display an overdeveloped superego. Siblings are supposed to get along and share together. Thus, we force the issue.

The strains of this fraudulent warmth are so great that, more often than not, we drink and self-medicate to numb the tension. It only gets worse with time. What to do?

Cut out the crap. As the saying goes, "You can choose your friends, but you're stuck with your relatives." The first half is correct; the second is a bunch of baloney. You don't like someone, you avoid them. Seem harsh? Listen—at this stage in your life, you don't need the STRESS. You shouldn't be forced to like someone by an accident of birth. (There. I've just alienated my parents and brother.) It took me a long time to say this out loud.

That doesn't mean you have to be antagonistic. Far from it. Help-out where you can. Be there for advice; a good listener is a gift to others. Remember the special occasions. Just don't go overboard when it's simply through 'obligation.'

I can't draw the line for you—or for me, either. You'll have to feel your way through. I think it'll be obvious when things get out-of-balance.

Now, there's one thing you might always share with your brother or sister—physical resemblance. This commonality will be pointed-out by others. (More often than not, you don't think you look at all alike.) What's interesting is that some say you look like this one; others like that one. And they're all adamant about their opinions. You'll find this mildly amusing. That's about it. The 'accident of birth thing,' again. Just surface similarities. Nothing to get all excited about.

The lesson here is stark and simple: if your brother wants to be an important part of your life, he needs to become a friend, first. He'll have to work on that and earn your friendship. Like anyone else. I'm sure you'll respond in kind. If not, write him off.

Do I have Adult A.D.D.?

Attention Deficit Disorder. Hmmm…..Kind of rolls off the tongue nice. It's now a commonly-recognized ailment of youth. Kids used to be behavior problems in the classroom; now they're cloaked in the guise of a syndrome which excuses being just plain bad by an inability to concentrate. And they're supposedly intelligent, to boot. Oh, God!! In any event, A.D.D.'s politically correct.

Guess what, guys? The psych establishment now says adults can suffer from the same malady. That's right, when we daydream or just fail to complete assigned tasks we're not to blame. We really WANT to get the job done. It's just that we're distracted by birds, beasts, women (or men), snacks, etc. And all this due to some chemical imbalance in the brain. Voilà!! No more responsibility. We'll just be treated and get back on the right track.

Want to know what I think? (a rhetorical question). This is bullshit. Blatant rationalization. An effort to perpetuate a value system we really don't want to be a part of, anymore.

We don't concentrate because we want to be somewhere else, doing something else.

Here's a litmus test to determine if you're really clinical or just frustrated:

Choose one:

A. I can't seem to get my tasks completed at work, and often find myself up against deadlines—even though I had months in advance to finish.
My disfunction is the result of:
   1. An inability to focus.
   2. Mental confusion.
   3. Too much sex the night before.
   4. Too little sex the night before.
   5. Daydreaming about the Coffee Shop.
   6. All of the above.

OK—that wasn't so bad. Let's try another one:

B. We're driving to the mall on a Saturday afternoon, and my wife (with animation) is relating the latest chapter in the long-standing feud between her Mom and Cousin Bunny. Sensing that I'm nodding but not listening, she confronts me and asks me to summarize the last 10 minutes. I tell her I agree—we haven't had such good weather in ages. I'm dead meat.
My disfunction is the result of:
   1. An inability to focus.
   2. Mental confusion.
   3. No sex since last month.
   4. No sex since last year.
   5. Thinking about which weapon to use.
   6. All of the above.

You're doing great! One more for good measure:
C. You've just been elected to Congress, and are about to give your first public speech, dedicating the Mary Louise Beauregard

Smith III Memorial Library. You memorized it, but have drawn a complete blank at the last moment. All you can remember are the words to 'Hey Jude.'
Your embarrassing disfunction is the result of:
1. An inability to focus.
2. Mental confusion.
3. Adopting Ronald Reagan as a role model.
4. Picturing Reagan having sex at 90.
5. Daydreaming about the Coffee Shop.
6. All of the above.

Pens down. You're finished.

If you've circled #1 and/or #2, your either lying, or you need immediate help. Proceed at once to the nearest emergency room!
Circling #s 3 and 4 are an easy fix: score some Viagra (for yourself or your mate).
However, if you consistently picked 5 or 6, you want to be somewhere else—doing something else. Sorry, there's nothing wrong with you that a saner life wouldn't solve.

So when you find yourself behind the office computer, struggling to stay on course while descending into a milky haze, take solace in this thought: your brain isn't self-destructing; its telling you to change. Heed the warning!

Looking Better…Younger…Slimmer…

Just returned from my local watering hole. Once a week I head over for drinks, a meal, and scoping the scenery. Recharges the old batteries, you know.

I wouldn't even think about taking my seat at the bar unless I looked good. Wait…translation: unless I THOUGHT I looked good. It's all in your head, pal.

When the hair's in place, and the shirt's just right, you look about the same to others as when you're out of whack. Ain't it a shame. With one big difference: 'looking' good means projecting good. And that's what makes the world go 'round.

How you think you appear inspires confidence, which bolsters your appeal. Self-confidence is acutely contagious.

Sophie

By anyone's definition, Sophie led a hard life. Every time the road looked good—there were obstacles strewn along the way. Even as a child.

She was the first daughter of a Jewish immigrant family from Hungary—though born in the States. Like many immigrants, her parents did what they could to provide for their children. They started their own business—a corner grocery store. Where—of course—everyone worked. And they stressed the value of education.

New Jersey winters weren't easy at the dawn of the 20th century. Sophie was fond of telling stories to illustrate the times: "Did I ever tell you about walking miles through the snow to go to the movies? This was my joy in life. As usual, my mother gave me the 2 pennies to buy a ticket." She paused for effect. "Well—after finally getting to the theater, I was told that tickets had gone up to 3 cents. So I walked all the way home for the extra penny, and then back again." In that story you catch a glimpse of the determination that was to guide Sophie throughout her long life.

She married late (over 30, though I'm not exactly sure) and never went to college. But Sophie had the family smarts, and was especially good with numbers. She took jobs as bookkeeper, accounting assistant, and secretary to a county court judge. Oh—she was particularly proud of that position. Yes—Sophie could excel in a man's world.

Sophie married a dashing young lawyer—a rogue cut from the Clark Gable mold. But before their first child was born, Sam was called to war. He fought on the front lines in France and Germany. He became a father in absence when their first child was born.

But Sophie was up to the challenge: "This isn't the first time I've been on my own."

Sam wrote letters, supposedly. On a regular basis, she would say. These kept her abreast of everything in his life—perhaps too much, as she could divine some womanizing on the side. In her typical manner, Sophie just dismissed this as men satisfying needs under extreme conditions. But she would talk endlessly about those letters—and how romantic they were, etc. Everyone would listen—true or not, the supposed existence of these letters was very important to her.

With the war over, the boys returned home and took up life with a vengeance. A son was soon born, a legal career established, home purchased near the park, booming times. Sophie's family entered the prosperous '50s enriched by children, family, friends, and the promise of a bigger and brighter future. It continued that way for awhile.

Until the MS hit. At first just an annoying twitch or numbness, Sam was diagnosed with multiple sclerosis in 1961. The case was particularly aggressive, and within a few years he became wheelchair bound. Sam's attitude didn't make it any easier. He fashioned himself as a tough guy in a Hemingway-kind of way. His verbal abuse couldn't help but take a toll on Sophie, even while attending to Sam's increasing physical needs.

And then there were the finances. Little income and increasing expenses. Rather than lose the home, Sophie dug deep-down and again rose to the challenges. She contacted her cousin in Washington, D.C. Ted was (and is) a brilliant man—and had many connections in and out of government. "I know Ted can do something," Sophie would say. Her faith in what education and raw intelligence could accomplish was unbendable.

She was right. Ted convinced the Army that the illness was "service-related." As a result of this determination, their home became tax-exempt—and government benefits flowed like running water.

Sophie did everything. She learned how to drive—and maintained her independence. Took her children here and there. Ran the household like clockwork. Kept Sam comfortable. She worked overtime to keep everything going .

But Sophie didn't stop there. She became a model volunteer. She gave what little extra time she had to her Temple Sisterhood. She worked as a bookkeeper for the Boys' Club. Helped her brother's law practice flourish. (I'm sure that you've heard stories like this before; this one is for real.)

Sam went in and out of Veteran's Hospitals with increasing frequency until he died in 1973 of a virulent staph infection. Sophie's life was to change again.

After twelve years of caring for an invalid husband, Sophie could now begin to live. And she did—to some degree. She took her first real vacation and went to Mexico. A few years later she traveled to Israel on a tour. Then it stopped.

Illness encroached again. This time it was her. Rheumatoid arthritis and diabetes set in.

She lost the desire to travel—and, instead, focused on her children and their families. Like always, she never-ever put herself first. She even found more time to volunteer—this time for the hospital auxiliary, which turned into a 20-year stint.

After Sophie turned 80, her family stood around in front of the house as her beloved car was driven away by its new owner. It was no longer safe for her to drive. She went downhill from that day forward.

Sophie suffered a slow and agonizing death. Her body shut down little-by-little in the last eight years. But she never left her home of 50 years until the last 3 months, when live-in-care was no longer adequate for her condition. Sophie's mental acuity never vanished—which was the final indignity. She was aware of her pain and predicament till the end.

Which came in February. She just slipped away during the night.

The house on Maple Street has new occupants—a young family with children. That would make Sophie very happy.

Before it was sold, her children gathered on a windswept day to take stock of its contents—to box-up the remnants of a life spanning 89 years. While rummaging through the garage, a packet of musty envelopes bundled together with string was found under the tool chest.

They were the letters sent by Sam during WWII. Throughout the day and night that followed, the children read every one and passed them around from one to another. The caring and love jumped right off the pages even after 60 years. I believe that the discovery of these letters was a final gift from their mother.

Sophie's life has taught me to search for that elusive happy medium: care for family and do what you can for all; but find the time to enjoy yourself. She never had that.

Being Charles Kuralt

I felt moved telling Sophie's story. (Seriously—no joking there.) But there's more to it than her tale alone.
Meeting ordinary people. Doing extraordinary things. In the most mundane of places. There's a mystical real-world quality to such encounters, indelibly etched into my psyche by the prosaic reporting of Charles Kuralt.
Charlie passed in 1997—a victim of complications brought on by treatment for lupus. I'm still mourning the loss.
Before his untimely death, I looked forward to each Sunday morning for 2 things: gorging on a 'Dutch Baby' at the local pancake house; and watching Charles Kuralt's reports on CBS. I figure there's got to be a connection somewhere. The easy answer would be the obvious resemblance between feeding my face and Kuralt's jolly girth. The deeper significance rests in wanderlust and simple truths.
Think I've envied the guy with the Porsche or the stud making it with a different babe every night?
Wrong.
I've been fascinated by (and more than a tad jealous of) Kuralt's journeys through backroad America. The mere thought of getting in a Winnebago and stopping at a greasy diner way down US 27 makes me horny. Schmoozing with the locals

would almost be too good to imagine.

I think it's about getting away from it all and connecting with others. Without being defined by who you are, what job you have, what station in life you've reached. Being able to converse on a variety of subjects and learning in response. Like being a kid in a candy store: each character you meet up with adding a new and tasty treat to the menu.

And, yet, there's the gnawing feeling that this sojourning exercise will come to an inevitable end with the realization 'there's no place like home.' Let me put it another way: the journey is one we have to take to cleanse ourselves and be free, only then to appreciate the fundamental idea of making one place—one special place—our own place.

But with a fresh understanding of where we fit into this picture and feeling secure with our piece of the puzzle. Without looking elsewhere.

Thank you, Charlie. I don't think you ever got to make that point. You surely intended to.

Being apologetic—sorry I've brought that up

I'm sorry. I'm sorry that I'm sorry. You can go on and on.

Here's an idea: start tomorrow morning, and count how many times you say this in the course of the day. I'll bet you run out of paper.

Our collective lack of self-esteem has reached the point that we've become the 'apologetic generation.' It's our fault that the world has problems.

I don't know about you, but I do this all the time—and it plum tires me out. I'm sorry you're not feeling well; I'm sorry that its raining ; Gee, I'm so sorry that you're late. OK, I'm convinced: I'm the root cause of all that's wrong. No more debate.

Truth is: we say "sorry" all the time, and no one really wants to hear it. But we're strangely compelled to apologize anyway. Now—all together, ask: "Why"?

Because society's beaten us down to a pulp. There's no tolerance for anything less than perfection: in character, in job performance, in personal relationships. Everyone looks for faultlines. Once seismically located, you take the blame. Doesn't matter how microscopically in error you might be—if it's wrong, you gotta take the heat. And you have to say: I'm sorry.

This is a bad habit, people. You have to go 'cold turkey' and

STOP THIS BEHAVIOR NOW!
Of course, such behavior modification will be a shock to your adversary-of-the-moment. Imagine the look on that face when you don't apologize for something you didn't do. The initial reaction will be to repeat the accusation—on the assumption that you didn't hear it the first time.

At this point, some deft maneuvering is called for. Your alternatives, in no particular order, are:

1. The Barrister Approach (follow a question with a question).
2. Rational Discussion (attempt to reason with your opponent).
3. Choke on an imaginary piece of meat (guaranteed to change the subject).

None of these are totally satisfactory solutions. But, generally speaking, they work.
Try them under appropriate circumstances.

Leaving the 'Sorry' world for a better one will bolster your self-esteem and earn others' respect. It will be a major league stress-buster, though not seeming so at the beginning. Once you overcome the fear of initial confrontation, the relief of not shouldering blame should be liberating. Even exhilarating.

It's a crucial step on the road to recovery.

I can't find a table at Barnes & Noble

Bookstores (and their obligatory cafes) have replaced supermarkets as our Main Street, Village Green, you name it. Excuse my ignorance, but for the life of me, I don't know how they stay in business.

On the one hand, they've replaced libraries—which now drain public funds while standing empty. In so doing, the bookstores are filled with readers doing what readers do—read. But they don't buy. That's why there're more shelvers than cashiers. Want a job there? Show the manager how many books you can carry under one arm.

On the other hand (and my pet peeve of the year), they've been transformed into study halls. Particularly the cafes. There's nothing more frustrating than savoring the anticipation of an evening with java and travel mag, only to be greeted by a sea of white notebooks. Filling every table and every chair. Which phenomenon, interestingly, stretches from September to June—coinciding with the school year. Hmm…

Ok—so I'll wait for a table.

Lots of luck! Two hours later (yeah-I timed it), the same faces were staring into the same notebooks at the same tables. Now, these kids are wise-asses. They buy one cup (cheapest thing on menu) and nurse it the whole night. No rules broken.

Can't be booted out.

After several repetitions, I decided to speak up. 'Speak-up'? No one's done that since the '60s. I did!!

Went to the cashier and complained nicely. Response: company regs don't allow us to interfere. Retort: I'd like to see the manager, please. Further response: the manager isn't here. But you can fill out this customer comment card, if you wish (she said, with a smirk on her face).

Grabbing a pen, I wrote down my opinionated rantings—and my well-thought-out suggestion. As follows: put up a small, though solicitous sign at the café entrance. It should read: "We know why you're here. Only to avoid being charged with discrimination, we'll tolerate you. But, PLEASE—try to stay only an hour. Thanks. Management."

"You" could mean anyone and everybody. Shzam!! No discrimination. Problem solved.

I was so proud of my idea, I e-mailed it the next morning to the parent company.

Via their 'customer relations' net address.

Naturally, I haven't had a reply. My idea's just too revolutionary. What a shame.

Because reading while sipping coffee is one of the true joys in life. Helps you clear out the cobwebs and stop time in its tracks. Caffeine's a mood-booster as well. And you learn something new along the way.

Just that it would be nice to sit down.

Design your own Talk Show

Now here's a fantasy as common as black leather and chains: being the host of your own talk show. Daytime or late night, whatever moves you. Think about it - and then make your dream come true!

Not possible? Not up to it? Don't know where to start? Don't think NBC would hire you?

Hey—you don't need the networks. Here's the plan:

1. Rent 'Wayne's World', and watch it.
2. Get a list of local-access cable channels.
3. Develop a topic. (*Seinfeld* aside, not even a double-digit cable station wants a show about nothing).
4. Spruce-up the outline with illustrations (stick figures will do).
5. Take the station manager out to a steak dinner.

The topic's the thing. No, don't waste time and energy coming up with some original idea. They're none left.

What you need is something boring. Programmers always like those. Isn't that obvious?

For example: a talk show about the weather, with musical guests. This is absolutely fascinating. Just think about it: you get to sit around and discuss the big events of the day—those monster midwest thunderboomers; F5 tornados; and even a Hurricane (that's for the two-hour specials!). You can invite guests—like those Weather Channel anchorpersons. They'd come. I know they're not booked on other shows.

And you'd never run out of material—'cause everyday the weather's new. You don't need to show repeats.

Not bad, right?

I think doing your talk show will refocus you away from daily strains and stresses. Then again, it might not. But you'd have to agree: it's a funny idea.

The Downside of Celebrity

Stay anonymous.

Infinitely better than trying to become famous. Or infamous (there's no difference).

Sometimes it seems that everyone wants their '15 minutes' of fame. Seriously, that's logical in our society. Every culture needs its nobility. Since we don't have princes and counts, we rank based on fame. The evidence is clear: *People Magazine* outsells *Time* exponentially.

We want to be recognized, written-about, treated royally, asked for autographs. Indeed, celebrity status is all that—but it's making a deal with the Devil.

I think you know what I mean in one sense: the loss of anonymity and privacy. Never being able to retreat into your own world , or just be yourself with family and close friends. But there's more to it than that.

Maintaining celebrity status is at the top of the stress 'Hit Parade.' Once you've had the taste of it—you fear its loss. Constantly. It permeates your life. You become defined by that last article or feature piece on the local news. If it only SEEMS to wane, you're on a downhill slide. In your mind. I should know.

In a prior life, I was a celebrated immigration attorney.

Appeared on NBC, CBS, ABC, and most of the other alphabet soups. Not to speak of *Time, USA Today, The New York Times, Washington Post*, and the *Miami Herald* on countless occasions. My sense of self depended upon appearing in print that day. If it didn't, I ceased to exist.

What a ridiculous life.

Well—maybe there's just a touch of sour grapes (my last article appeared over three years ago). But I'm better off without it. I can define myself by something other than recognition. Because you can't win that game.

So stick to your one-on-one circle of friends and acquaintances. Your affirmation of self can come from interaction with them. And not from your name in a newspaper. Just trust me on this.

All Life Stems from the 'Schmata' Business

Tell me, please: What is it about clothing?

I mean, it does serve practical and indispensable purposes—like keeping you warm in winter, and covering-up your genitals.

The mystery is style, exclusivity, and…price. What other product can you name that costs hundreds for a simple piece of cotton (or polyester, for that matter)? And what about the fools who trip over each other to pay it? No wonder our economy is built on a pile of spandex and designer jeans.

Yep—the clothing industry stole the fundamental precept of the car business: planned obsolescence. It's the only thing that keeps it going. And we support it—blindly. (Take a look at your last Visa bill). Come on, people, there's little sense in going bankrupt just to look good. I have a solution.

Recycle! If you hold onto a garment long enough, it comes back into style. Well—maybe not Nehru jackets. But just about everything else.

Look, I've got a closet full of narrow ties. So thin I feel like Roy Rogers putting them on. After years collecting dust, they now qualify for GQ. I'm going to wear them.

Here's another item: shoes. Dust 'em off, get some new heels ($5.00), and do the polish thing. New! Better than new—at least they look broken-in; there's nothing more gauche than showing-up in brand-new shoes that don't look worn at least once.

And then, of course, there's jeans. Actually, style now favors the 'worn' look. Can you beat that? My 20 year-old Levi's that shed are more 'in' than the new ones at Macy's. Jackpot! I can either wear them, or sell them on the Cuban black market. Win/Win.

So—what is it about clothing? I'll tell you: beat the system and save some money. More pennies for the Coffee Shop.

How to Survive a Singles Event

It's so exciting, and a bit intimidating. You've picked the singles "event" to zero-in on, and now the preparations are underway. Get ready for what will either be a great night—or major stress. Guys (and girls), it's all how you approach it!

Guess what? I've got a list of do's and don'ts:

I. Do:
1. Look Good.
2. Act Confident.
3. Don't get dressed until the time it starts.
4. Have a drink before you go.
5. Bring plenty of cash.

II. Don't:
1. Overdress.
2. Think too much (i.e., no agenda).
3. Arrive early.
4. Go with a friend.
5. Drink yourself into oblivion.

You want to be confident? You got to look good. Now—that's easy for some people; not for others (like me). There's no shortcut: it takes major training, big time.

Let's break it down. You got body, skin, and hair. Three elements. Each one gets a separate regimen. Skin and hair take less effort—so let's tackle body shape.

Ready? Take a deep breath, and go to the mirror. (Full-length, please). Don't suck it in. Now... look!

I'll bet you couldn't gaze for more than five seconds before turning away. Not a pretty sight. OK—suck it in. Well, not much improvement.

Start from scratch. Have the vision to see how you want to look, and get to it.

Use the fruit test: you look like a pear, right? Turn the pear upside down. That's how you should look. To do this, you need to build the shoulders, pecs, and upper arms; while cutting-out the carbs which feed that belly. It's not too difficult. Those pushups, twice a day on alternate days, will work wonders—IF you do them religiously. Don't miss a single session. Meanwhile, no bread (sigh) and no sweets. If you cheat, G-d will give you 2 lbs. and 2 inches for every slice. Trust me on this. It comes off with hard work, but comes back with just a nod.

Do this, and you'll be ready to roll in a month. Bide your time; it'll be worth it. Girls don't want pears; they want hunks. (OK: semi-hunks.) Don't believe their bullshit about the 'inner man.' Now...

Get dressed, man. I like black. No freakin' idea why it works, but it looks great. Ready?

It's Showtime!! (cue the music—Stayin' Alive works well)

You look great; you feel great; and you're on top of the world! For about five minutes.

Something's wrong. It's not working.

No one meets your gaze; or they avert it. Everyone else is

getting hit on, or doing the hitting. With apparent success. You've got a drink, a barstool, and—nothing.

Advice from that guy: stick with it. Keep going to these 'events.' You know what's happening? You're learning a language. Sooner or (like me) later, it starts to click. Like you're suddenly in sync with the crowd. It just happens. Confidence.

Then you'll ease-into those one-on-one conversations. Whether you follow-up or not, it'll be an enriching experience. Just manage your level of expectations.

And your drinking. Man, that's a killer. (literally). The singles world is centered around drinking—it's what finances the industry. You have to consciously resist. Have one; nurse it; and then switch to Sprite. If you don't, you'll feel and look like shit in short order. (And so will your wallet - $8 a drink adds up.)

We've been digressing. Where are we?

Oh yeah—do's and don'ts. In conclusion, there's one thing more than anything else you need when riding the singles circuit: cash; and lots of it. DO have it. If you don't, sorry. Don't venture out till you're flush. There's no point in surfing the scene without financial security. If you hit-it-off with someone, then what?

Enjoy those 'singles events'. If you're ready—mentally, physically, and financially. And only then. But you probably won't follow my advice. So enjoy the ride anyway while it lasts.

P.S.: Younger vs. Older Women*

*[Girls, you can skip to the next topic (unless you want to see how we men think. We do think, you know). It's just that I can't write about older/younger men—it's not within my hetero realm of experience]

Being just shy of the big '5-0' and immersed in crisis, you would think I'd be out hunting bimbos. The 20-30 types with endless legs and toned midriffs. Not me. Not interested.

In the ultimate of ironies, these young girls are only too eager to talk to (if not outright hit on) me. And all I see is my daughter's head pasted on their hardbodies.

No—I like the older ones. 40's—even 50's. More worldly and knowing; and with similar generational tastes - music; pop culture; music; art; music. More experienced (use your imagination). And not out to conquer the world.

Give me an older woman anytime. It just feels right—soothing, calm, not intimidating.

With one proviso:

Watch-out for the ones that never married and with a string of failed relationships. They're like "Black Holes"—they'll suck you in and drain your inner being.

OK—so how do you spot a Black Hole?

Fortunately, they haven't yet developed stealth technology. Here are the readily evident signs:

A. Their eyes stay focused on you like hot coals (I don't even think they blink);

B. They're incredibly accomplished conversationalists;

C. They initiate contact deftly, using any conceivable pretext; and

D. They never, ever, talk about themselves.

In other words, they make it **TOO EASY**. (Keep repeating the phrase to yourself—too easy, too easy, too easy.)

Let me give you an example. True story; just happened last week.

As is my custom, I'm sitting at the bar, cruising in my comfort zone at the weekly 'singles event' (see prior discussion). I'm in the mood to just scope the scenery.

About two hours-in, I get a tap on the shoulder. Turning around, a rather attractive brunette smiles and launches into this tirade. She asks, rather rhetorically: "Why do I attract such jerks?"

Now I'm thinking, this is one creative line. I'll play along. Burns and Allen time. George asks: "Why do you say that, Gracie?"

Without missing a beat, she responds: "This guy won't believe me, can you beat that? What a jerk!"

OK. So far so good. I'll continue playing straight man: "Believe you about what, dear?"

"That Michael Jordan wanted to date me."

This is getting real good. "Why wouldn't he believe you? I do." (You know, I actually think I did.)

"Yeah," she continued, "I went to school with him at Chapel Hill; Michael always said he wanted to date me."

George: "I'm sure he did. I agree; this guy's a jerk."
Gracie: "I like you, George."

That's it. In the next five minutes, she sucks in everything she needed to know about me. Her finely-tuned intuition tells her I'll oblige. Which, of course, I did—given the opportunity to talk about myself. I left that evening with her name and phone numbers on a napkin. And two other pieces of information: her occupation (nurse), and habitat (Boynton Beach). She knows my life story.

I haven't called her. Good boy. One less victim for her collection.

I'm learning.

Black Holes aside, older, mature women have it all. Soft around the edges while confident; demanding where it counts.

My therapist just e-mailed me a piece on older women by Andy Rooney. He says once you get by a few wrinkles, it only gets better from there on. As usual, Andy's right on the money.

Go see for yourself.

Art Shows....

...are not for Art. Surprised? (I don't think so.)
 In Florida, these shows proliferate during the "season" (i.e., winter months). Usually relegated to weekends—so the paycheck-earners have an excuse to blow some bucks.
 If you go to more than one or two, you'll realize that there's nothing new. It's the same traveling roadshow. Same booths; same artists; same shit. The only things missing are the circus train and bigtop.
 But—every Saturday and Sunday—they're out there in droves, walking this endless circle five abreast. Hardly anyone buys anything. Why DO they go?
 Can't be the food: funnel cakes and kilbasa (*sic*) really don't merit a $10 parking fee. And can't be the weather: it's always too windy, hot, cold, whatever.
 I finally figured it out yesterday. People go 'cause it's free!!
 Americans will go anywhere. Stand on endless lines; fight crowds; pay for parking and junk food—all because the main event is free.
 'Art Shows' are a classic example.
 It just gets to me that people don't buy anything. I can only wonder how those journeymen artists cover their expenses. The only conceivable explanation is that they're independently

wealthy by night, starving artists by day. That's it!! The 'shows' are their schmooze-mobiles. Their 'coffee shops.' I envy them, folks—they've made it to the Promised Land, and I'm still waiting.

For us mortals, though, the deeper secret to these shows is that they provide an alternate venue for an ever-growing sport: people watching. Europeans have been doing this forever, starting with and sustaining the outdoor café industry. They simply grab a seat in a chic locale (say, Venice's St. Marks square), and gaze at the beautiful people on parade. Everyone wins: the gazers get to feed their fantasies, and the paraders have their egos stroked. The attractors and the atractees. It's as old as Adam and Eve. It's safe; it's acceptable; and its....free!

Of course, being Americans, we're way behind and only slowly emerging from our puritanical shells. But we're catching on. Think those Beaneries and Starbucks litter the sidewalks for caffeine alone? Wrong! They're our first vehicles for sipping while watching the Main Street parade.

Art Shows are a start. Until people stroll to be noticed (without any pretext), the shows fill that void. It's something we need, simply because it makes us feel better. Because it's stimulating.

There's nothing wrong with that. And remember: it's cheap.

Playing the Piano

I'm a talented piano-player. For real! Can play by ear, even though trained. I should have done that for a living. But you know how that goes (nice Jewish boy needs a profession…).

I started taking lessons at 6. Not atypical in the '50s. My Mom was perceptive—figured that a non-athletic type with nerdish tendencies needed something. She was right.

Being musical is the one constant in my life.

It's always cropping-up at every corner. Like right now. I'm in this mood to attack a classical piece. Yeah…Chopin comes to mind. For the sense of accomplishment. Besides, its nice to use your talent, once in awhile.

I have a theory: that playing some musical instrument alters your brainwaves. Kind of like electric shock therapy—but more mellow (I would hope so). I seem to recall an article someplace about 'golgi bodies'—or something like that. Exercising a different part of your head. I remember, now. Musicians' develop differently, in the cerebral context. So says the AMA.

It's probably true. After I play for 30 minutes, I feel different. It's hard to quantify, but it goes something like this: play Sinatra, and you feel like swinging. Play Chopin, you think culturally. Play Ray Charles—and the sky's the limit!! (He's my favorite.)

Rhythm. All music has it, in one style or another. But, hey—

people have a rhythm, too. Some call them 'moods', but it's really rhythm. And playing music can alter it.

Better yet—it's not expensive, and it's not a controlled substance.

You don't have to be great at it. All you have to do is try.

However (bet you knew that was coming), once one masters the piano, guitar, piccolo, slide trombone—you're on call 24/7. Whether you like it or not. There's nothing worse.

Typical example:

Dinner parties. At someone's home.

If you play the piano, and they know it, watch out. You're the show.

First thing to do is case the house upon arrival. Upon spying a piano, develop a locktight excuse before they ask.

Having been through this on myriad occasions, I've got some that always work:

1. Before sitting down for cocktails, announce offhandedly: "What a week! My arthritis has been acting up".

2. Pre-empt the hosts by playing your latest atonal composition.

3. Pull out your exclusive contract with Steinway . (Trust me—they don't have a Steinway.)

4. Choke on a piece of meat.

As great as music is, it's a disaster when you're not in the mood. Never play under those circumstances. Play when you're ready. When you're psyched. It's an elixir.

Incidentally, as an aphrodisiac, you can't beat it. You'll see!

The Sounds of Silence

No book about reducing stress is complete without a discourse on the benefits of noise elimination. So let's tackle it.

I'm convinced, at age 49, that I suffer from a mild hearing loss. Nothing severe—but enough to be uncomfortable for me and annoying to others.

I know what caused it.

Too many years of TV shouting at me, cars and trucks belching away, and—of course - loud music, have taken its toll. I'm absolutely amazed that all the old 'rockers' aren't stone deaf as well as wasted.

Try "quiet" for a day—or a week, if you can manage it. At first, it will drive you crazy. Stick with it.

You'll soon descend into a slow, silky haze. Well…not actually a haze. Because your thinking process will become less cluttered—and more focused. It's amazing!

That's the nice thing about getting out of bed early, and walking or writing (like now). It's quiet. Soothing. You can actually get things done. Or you can just think. No intrusions.

It's addictive. Bad word, I know. But getting up early is a treat. You won't stop. And you don't do it out of necessity—you do it for the quiet. It's so easy.

The real trick is how to bring quiet to your day-in-progress (like the 9-to-5 section). If you can do that, I think you're well on to mastering your daily life. Just let me know how. I need it.

Coincidences…

…are not really coincidences. At least that's Boyer's Theory #23.

See, I believe in fate. It goes with my maternal-side ancestry. They're supposed to be from a long line of Jewish witches and healers. Really. So I'm receptive to the unknown. The fact that I can't explain it logically doesn't diminish my faith.

I never thought about coincidences in the same league as Ghostbusters before this past week. Since Wednesday (its now the following Monday), almost every day has brought on a coincidental occurrence. Must be a sign. (Twilight Zone music time.)

Here's the rundown:

Wednesday: My daughter (at college) has a dream involving my mother crying, and breaking bottles against a wall. Coincidence: my brother started drinking again earlier that night, and my parents had to bring him back to their place to dry out.

Thursday: I drive up to Boca to a 'start-the-weekend-early' singles event. Strike up a conversation with a guy my age. Coincidence: went to summer camp with him 35 years ago. Second coincidence: My therapist (remember Kathy?) shows up with her girlfriend in tow. The girlfriend is his ex-fiance.

Friday: Finally get together with a guy I met several weeks back. He lives in Jersey, and comes down like twice a year. Arthur. Very likeable. He asks what I've been up to (meaning: who am I seeing, etc.). I tell him. He smiles. Says he dated her last summer when he was down for a week. Absolutely amazing. I mean, what are the chances of this? Except that:

On Sunday: I go to a mixer only two blocks (miraculously) from my office. No brainer. Sit down at the bar next to Steve, an accountant for the City of Miami. You guessed it. Dated same girl a month ago. Described her to a "t."

    Of course, I could approach all this scientifically. I could call Arthur. He's a professor of statistics. We could draw a graph.
    I don't think so. I prefer to view all this as a parapsychologic or spiritual episode. You can't prove it isn't.
    I need to view it all as spiritual. That's a fact. It reminds me that I can't control everything in my life.
    Voodoo and miracles aside, it's important to give up the 'control' thing. There's just so much you can do to keep life in order. At some point, you have to shrug your shoulders and just accept fate. Shit happens. You can't avoid all of it.
    After last week's events, I'm more receptive to this theory. Yeah—you can (and probably should) stay disciplined. Do the prudent things. To a point. Then, let the chips fall where they may—because they're going to, anyway.
    Again, you can't control everything. (I'm being repetitive because this is really important). I suspect that accepting this proposition is a major stress-buster. There's nothing to lose by trying.

How to Relax Without Drinking

It CAN be done! But you've got to employ certain tricks and sleight-of-hand. The idea is to look like you're drinking—when in reality, you're not.
I have some creative ideas. Here we go:

1. Order a club soda on the rocks.
Upside: If you can stomach paying 3 bucks for a 50-cent can, this is by far the best way to fake it. Usually it's a tall glass, so you can nurse it for an hour. Besides—it looks like Absolut. Want to sweat the details? Have 'em add a slice of lime for effect.
Downside: Too many bubbles. Make sure you cover your mouth when you burp. And deep-six the straw.

2. Ask for a glass. Just a glass.
Upside: Costs nothing. Looks real if you hold it with a napkin.
Downside: Looks stupid if you sip from it.

3. Offer to buy a drink for someone else.
Upside: You look like a "pro"—real classy; and gracious at the same time. By the time they finish their drink, they won't

even notice you're abstaining.
Downside: Unless you're the designated driver, your motives are questionable.

4. Say you arrived early and had your quota.
Upside: Makes sense. Anyone getting someplace too early will start drinking out of sheer boredom. Also shows a responsible attitude—knowing when to stop.
Downside: When the bartender asks if you're finally ready for one.

Now that you've got your agenda, put it into action. Problem is, you're going to get sidetracked. Don't be discouraged.
Here's what's likely to happen:
You'll have your first drink and get 'in the mood.' The buzz feels good, and a bit more would be just right. "Pour me another Absolut," he says, with an air of familiarity. And so on.
That's the critical point. If you have that second drink, pay and…walk out. Because the third one is just around the corner, and now you have no willpower. When you come back next week, try the one drink exercise again. And again. Until you get it right.
Otherwise, its all downhill. Trust me (again) on this.
I have an alcoholic brother. I've seen the weakness at work. It's not funny.
Remember Dean Martin? Dean made drinking-to-excess funny and cool for an entire generation. (Like sliding down a brass pole till he landed at the bar.) That's our downfall. We've internalized this value system. Don't ask Dean, though—he's dead.
Abstaining doesn't mean you're a Puritan. Or worse, a nerd. It's just a good way to stay healthy and alive. And save some

money.

If that's too much of a switch for you, try the virtual approaches noted above. But please—just one drink.

Club Soda forever!!

Visiting Fantasy Island

Contrary to your darkest fears, you're not the only one with fantasies. We all have'em.

Fess up: When you hear "de plane, de plane," don't your palms start to sweat? Come. Mr. Rourke beckons you.

We love our fantasies. Which we keep to ourselves, for fear of being either Baker-acted or arrested for lewd and lascivious behavior. The thing is—you're not alone. And I think they're kind of healthy. At least interesting.

So—we're dealing with 2 types: grandiose and sexual. Getting excited? Think I'm about to get into X-rated stuff?

OK—taboos and family embarrassments aside (like if my daughter reads this), here goes:
Sex fantasies first.

I'm going to tell you a few of mine—but we'll get to that in a minute. We need to start-off with some general discussion..

I think we fantasize, sexually, to escape our everyday world. That's what happens to me. For at least 10-20 minutes, I'm somewhere else doing something exciting—with no stress or consequences. It's as exciting—and risk-free—as I desire. Could be at night; and often during the day. Doesn't have to involve masturbation (though it often does).

More than physical release—it gives me some separation

from the mundane anxieties which never end (e.g.: work; bills; chronic responsibilities). Then I feel refreshed. The 'ole "recharge the batteries" routine.

Here are a few of my recurring themes:

1. Tall women. Always been attracted to them, but not sure why. Usually white women—and thin. I like to compare them to myself. (You'll have to use your imagination from here on).
2. Short women. Not as frequent, and rather new on the block. Still white thin ones.
Same deal: body comparisons. Usually in sexual situations.
3. Older women. (Sorry, people—no kinky same-gender stuff in my repetoire). The most recent addition to the collection. Certainly the most sophisticated. Picturing them lose their control and turn animalistic. Really gets me going.

Something tells me yours are different. It doesn't really matter much. Whatever gets those juices flowing serves the purpose.

(*Incidentally: please contact me. I'm starting to collect an anthology of sex fantasies for my next book. If you want to be included, here's your chance. More details to come.)

Now—for the Grandiose fantasies.
Some might call them 'delusions of grandor.' That's a pet-phrase in clinical psychology. I don't like the word 'delusion.' Implies you're crazy. "Fantasy" sounds more like a sci-fi flick. More acceptable.

The situations vary sharply, but with one prevailing similarity: you—the dreamer—are central to an unfolding drama. Usually involving some issue of importance. Could be political intrigue. Often can be a hero/heroine situation. Might even involve family gatherings.

What I find is that you prove you're better than people realized. Let's rephrase that. The fantasy is a boost to your self-esteem.

Here's one of my favorites:

Remember *The Verdict* starring Paul Newman? Well, it's kind of the same thing, but I'm playing the Newman role. (Frank whatever that last name is.)

I'm a washed up attorney (very true), who once was at the top of the crop (also true). Doing menial briefs/cases for a check. Until—one day—there's this client that deserves better in life. And the juices start to flow.

The old creativity and energy get cranking. It keeps getting better from there on, culminating in one big, final court hearing. I rise from counsel table, and slowly—deliberately—give the best speech of my life. There's not a dry eye in the house. The client wins. Everyone lives happily ever-after.

I love it!! Yeah—its just a game. Inside my head. But it wisks me away to a better place—if only for a brief interlude.

Fantasies are a necessity for the war-weary. Are they healthy? Well now, what's better: satisfying hallucinations; or cardiac arrest from too much reality?

My friend, the answer to this question may color the rest of your life.

Quitting Smoking

I'm on day three. I know I'm really trying this time, having nearly killed an innocent bystander this morning. Didn't like the way she looked at me.

Few challenges facing modern man are more daunting than quitting cigarettes. Once nicotine digs its claws in, you lose control over life.

Smokers uniformly suffer from a fundamental misconception: that smoking reduces stress and anxiety. Sadly, this is a delusion. About the only thing a good cigarette does is soothe a momentary craving. Period. The rest is all suicidal.

OK, fellow puffers. Let's think this through. First, we'll list all the negatives about smoking:

1. Harms your health.
2. Saps energy.
3. Yellows your teeth.
4. Wrinkles your skin.
5. Makes you smell like an old car.
6. Makes you look like a moron.
7. Turns-off the opposite sex (unless they happen to be smokers also—the worst thing that can happen to you).
8. Costs the equivalent of a good vacation a year.

And the positives:
1. Five minutes of relief.

Considering the state of the world today, it's absolutely no surprise that for millions of otherwise intelligent people - the positive outweighs the negatives. No surprise at all.

It's time to step-up and be tested: Do YOU have the strength to throw them away? Without cheating?

Unless you're God-like, you're going to need some help.

Forget patches, hard candies, hypnosis, even cold turkey. I've got some fresh ideas:

Date a Non-smoker. This shouldn't be too difficult. It's getting harder to find a partner who smokes, anyway.

If you want to continue the relationship, you'll be forced to quit. Why? Because you can't hide it. Impossible. I've tried every trick there is: washed my mouth out with soap; fumigated my clothes; hid the pack in restrooms and under the floor mat of the car; etc. Give it up; they know. It's in the hormones.

You want a social life? Take the course of least resistance. Don't smoke.

Get active in a Church or Synagogue. A great idea. But you got to get real active. Spend a lot of your time there, and there'll be no opportunity to smoke. In any event, smoking on holy ground would be sacrilegious.

Get a job on the 30th floor. You have to smoke outside at work. That means elevator rides all day long. By the time you get down there, the craving will pass. Either that, or your boss will wonder where you've been all day.

Of course, if none of that works, you can always jump out

the window.

Remove all Stress from your life by Relocating to an Island in the South Pacific. This'll do it, for sure. No phones; no clients; no schedule; no problems. No need to smoke.

No money? Go back to the first three.

Whatever the method, you've got to stop smoking. Not tomorrow—today. You probably won't get as anxious, which'll make life easier.

You'll be saving money, too. $4 a pack is 28 bucks a week. And you know what that means: more towards the Coffee Shop!

Job Security: the endless quest!

'Job Security' doesn't exist. It's as extinct as dinosaurs. As phony as a $3 bill. As available for purchase as the Brooklyn Bridge.

Unless you work for the Federal Government (they're afraid to fire anybody), your job is good for today only. Tomorrow is a bonus. I think you all feel what I mean.

What in hell has happened? Used to be that a big company took care of you for life. The bigger and bluer the chip, the more secure the job. Seems to be just the opposite now.

No wonder the 30-somethings move from company to company every other year. They know.

This is one instance where my parents' advice has failed. The 'greatest' generation grew up believing that a job with General Motors or IBM was like a gilded cocoon. Unfortunately, that evaporated sometime in the '80s. For financial reasons best known to them, today's Dow Jones giants control their costs by continually adjusting their workforce. Better accept this reality. It's not about to change.

So—what shall we do?

Good conservative advice would have you work for yourself, or for a small, but growing firm where everyone knows your name. However…

There're some other approaches.

If you've got brass balls, you can employ the 'J. Edgar Hoover' insurance plan. Very simply, that's where you maintain a dossier on supervisors and upper management. Intercepted communications are good; compromising photographs even better. You can let them know what you know at appropriate times. You'll either get what you want or end-up at the bottom of the river. High stakes. Be careful.

Or: Adopt a 24/7 work schedule. Show the boss how extraordinary you really are. This avenue is only to be implemented under emergent circumstances. Like if big layoffs are coming. Be ready to kiss your social life goodbye. And realize that you've raised the bar—they'll expect the same or more from that point on.

The better road is to plan ahead while you still have your job. Make a solid, albeit small investment. Conservative is best. Nurture it weekly, if not daily. You need your 'safety net' and gameplan for that rainy day. It's gonna come.

Comedians & Comedy

My former fiance says I'm NOT funny. This was the constant theme in our relationship. Probably why it ended.

Might as well have said I have a grotesque facial deformity. You see, society places a well-developed funnybone near the top of the wish list. If you've got it—the sacred "sense of humor"—you've got it made!

Here's one instance where conventional wisdom is right on target. Funny IS better! And funny is healthy. That's why the best comedians live—and live well—on into their 90s. It's no coincidence.

George Burns (he lived to 100) was the best ever. Hands down. We'll use him as our laboratory rat. Let's dissect:

Issue: What made George funny?

Flip Answer: Flawless timing and an ability to remember ridiculous songs.

Reflective Answer: An indefinable, uniquely personal talent. You can't learn to be funny, in the truest sense. Either you're funny or not. And if you're not—forget it. Go on to something else.

But if you've got "it"—flaunt it. Revel in the glow. Because you're one of the chosen people. A word of advice, though—just don't put too much effort into the exercise.

Did you ever notice how painful it is watching someone *try* to be humorous? The thing that made "Saturday Night Live" so awful throughout the '90s was that it *tried too hard.*
Bits went on way too long. Pratfalls begot pratfalls, ad nauseam. Slapstick reigned supreme.

Lorne Michaels and crew lost track of a basic truth: comedy is a minimalist art. It's analogous to dancing: slight movement is graceful; exaggerated steps suggest two left feet.

Nuances. (What an intriguing word.) 'Funny' has to be incidental. You can't LOOK like you're attempting to be funny. Really. A raised eyebrow; simple staring; an occasional stammer. These work. Again, refer back to George Burns. While Gracie bantered-on about her sister's nonsensical exploits, George would just glance over towards the audience. Hilarious. No falls, no jokes. Just a look.

Now that you know what's humorous and what's not, employ it in your everyday life. Watch it diffuse confrontation and dissolve stress.

And don't worry if it doesn't always work. Mel Brooks (amongst others) throws out a gag-a-minute. At least one in every ten score. He aims for the law of averages.

The worst that can happen is you'll get a pie in your face. But even that can be funny. Just ask Soupy Sales.

You Can't Control Everything—Ouch!!

What I'm really talking about is that feeling of "Being in Control." The Jewish woman's nirvana. That elusive—and fraudulent—goal. It's the source of most earthly misery. At best, you'll come close. But , I guarantee, you won't get there.

Listen up: if you don't purge the fixation, you will NEVER be happy.

Let go.

It's a classic desensitization process. That's right—just like a fear of flying or creepy, crawly spiders. Clinical psychology 101.

Translation: take one step at a time. Little baby ones, for now. You gotta go slow; otherwise, you'll freak-out. Like you're free-falling through a bottomless mine shaft.

The thing is, you must find a fool-proof starting point.

I've got one:

Go camping in the Florida Everglades for 3 days. You heard me. To the capital of airboats and land of giant mosquitoes. Where the only compass is the stars above you.

Lie back and look up. Empty your head and merge with the heavens. See how constant they are. Let yourself go. Surrender to the universe.

Then look around you; take stock. You're still there; and

still intact. You're nothing but a speck in the scheme of things. Able to control nothing. But you're OK. Repeat the exercise for reinforcement.

The Everglades jaunt is good (just remember to bring a citronella candle). If you can't get there, or you're not all that ambitious, you can try 'screaming.' Or what's commonly called Primal Therapy.

What does this accomplish other than disturbing the peace?

It lets it all out. Purges the system. Burns the excess energy. When you're finished, you won't even have the strength to worry. You'll also have a sore throat.

The point is: Life's too short to worry; to try and get a handle on uncontrollable situations. So stop now. Listening? Or are you just being polite?

Giving-up the Snickers Bar

While you can't and shouldn't even attempt to control events, the flipside applies to what you put in your own body. Especially the packaged, manufactured junk that tastes so good—but converts you into processed swiss cheese.

At the top of this disreputable heap sits that vaunted symbol of desire—the royalty of all candy—the Snickers Bar. Displayed in all its regal splendor behind the museum glass of a nearby vending machine. It's calling to me now…"Bob, come get me. I'm yours."

Today, I succumbed to the seduction. My willpower is just too minor league to offer resistance. The Devil's work is clearly at play here. It's insidious.

No folks, the genius of American technology was not sending a man to the moon and back. True genius was creating the Snickers Bar. From the graphic design, to the feel of the wrapper, to the texture of the chocolate outer-layer. What an exercise in human understanding. They nailed it!

Even the anticipation of getting x into z (translation: bar into mouth) is pleasure incarnate. I love the ritual of slowly tearing open the wrapper until the chocolate shows through. The smell wafts over about two seconds later. No human can resist it.

Then comes the first bite. A big one. All that chocolate and caramel overloading the senses. The rush is equivalent to Niagara.

Of course, what goes up, must come down. Two hours later I want another one. And so forth. All this keeps the economy pumping and America great.

And that's what's wrong. What's great for our nation (sound the trumpets!!) is bad for Bob. Intellectually, I understand. But put the Snickers in front of me, and it's history.

Seriously—as we age, we have to treat our bodies better. Unless you want to encourage a chronic illness. If, however, you want to stay healthy, keep away from the chemicals and eat natural. It will cost a bit more, but it's worth it.

This is not meant to be an ideological statement. It's just the truth.

Portal-Potties and the Kabbalah

An introduction is necessary.

I headed up to Gainesville (Florida) this past weekend to visit with my daughter. At the University of Florida (UF, if you please). Rather than a mere lunch-dinner-breakfast scenario, my son and I attended lectures and poetry readings sponsored by the Hillel society. Topic: Judaism and Eastern spirituality. Or, trying to meld one with the other.

Turned a visit into an experience.

Mixing Buddhist theology with being Jewish—at first blush—seemed a bit over the top. Let's call it an 'academic exercise.' Especially when Allen Ginsburg was mentioned. He's like the mandatory Kevin Bacon of the University circuit—appearing, at least by reference, in every intellectual setting.

Then I got interested. And it wasn't just a recounting of the Dalai Llama dialoguing with learned rebbe's that finally caught my ear. It was the idea—no, the reality—of the soul.

Although I've had glimpses of a secondary consciousness throughout my life, I ascribed them to déjà vu or some other psych phenomenon. That's the product of a Western mind steeped in rationality.

This past weekend, I realized it might be something else.

I'll tell you how I connected. You're definitely going to laugh.

But it's true!

Portal-potties. (i.e., the john as a personal Stargate). It just clicked in my head. For almost as long as I can remember, going back to grade school, I've had this periodic but rare thought. Simply, that time had passed since the last time I had the thought that time had passed; but I remained the same. A constant. And observing—just observing—this passage of time in my life.

These thoughts only occurred while on the john. It still happens. Might be two years between 'events,' or as many as five. But its always the same. The me that notes time passage never seems to have changed. It watches the 'outer' me, and just takes stock.

Could this be my soul? A rip in space or time allowing it to surface and look around?

This is a cosmic happening in my otherwise workaday life. Somehow, I'm connecting to another me. I'm convinced: it's definitely out there. Nearby. Watching and waiting.

And a glorious sense of peace—even eternity—is enveloping me as I write about it. Here's what I feel: there is no time; there is only my own consciousness and a supreme being. That consciousness, like G-d, never ages. Beyond that is beyond me.

Back to the weekend.

Around us were students and faculty that studied (or were in the process of studying) Kabbalah. Jewish mysticism/ spirituality. Trying to bring spiritualism into mainstream Judaism. Or at least into Jewish lives.

I can't tell you about it—as I haven't read anything, yet. It's at the top of my list, however. (Before Stephen King.) Because Western society, as we know and experience it, produces no sense of self. Only stress and anxiety.

So I had a wonderful weekend in more than one way. Let's see where it all goes from there.

Guys & Dolls (Not the Show; as in Friendship)

Guys and girls can't be 'just friends'. It's one of our fondest wishes. But it just ain't meant to be.

For the last 4 weeks I've embarked on (for me, at least) a novel experiment: having a girl friend (as opposed to girlfriend). Verrrry interesting…

Getting straight to the point: it doesn't work. Other than pleasantries and shared war stories with fellow employees, heterosexual male/female friendships (the platonic type) just don't last. For a variety of reasons.

The first being incompatible intentions. Rather, feelings. One party usually wants things to heat-up; the other, happy to keep it at arm's length.

That leads to possessiveness and—here it comes—jealousy. Then you're sucked-in. Backing-off is going to hurt somebody.

Lets's say you try the friendship idea, anyway. At least be on the watch for:

A. Being on a phone "schedule." (or getting calls during the workday.)

B. Seeing him/her more than once a week.

C. Spending more than you should.

D. Not seeing other people (goes for either party).

E. Sex. (NOT a good idea.)

If you can avoid not just one, but every item listed above, you're OK—for now. But you're still sitting on a ticking bomb.

How many emotional explosions and bad break-ups do you need to experience before it all sinks in?

Don't hang around with the opposite sex unless you're willing to get involved. I had to be reminded of that yesterday. So I'm terminating my 'experiment.' It won't work; and it's not fair.

I realized she was upping-the-ante. What tipped-me-off? What you might call a 'float the trial balloon' scenario. Says she: "My therapist warns me that I'm not ready for a relationship." Idiot male that I am, I take that at face value. It seems safe.

I'm an idiot because she means just the opposite. Just testing me, my reactions, and convincing herself (out loud) to do the reverse.

And in the next five minutes, she assumes we'll go out to dinner on Saturday (even picks the restaurant); plans another prior get-together before the weekend (so we can get high). Totally contradictory.

Again, stupid male. It took a good day for all the above to sink-in. She doesn't want a friendship—she wants the whole enchilada. What's worse, she's still coming off an old relationship, and can't stop talking about the guy. I'm her vehicle for getting over him.

I didn't waste any time, and applied the brakes. She probably hates me now and thinks I've met someone else. Couldn't be farther from the truth.

I hope she reflects back and realizes that I really wanted a friend. That while I admitted an attraction to her, this wasn't what motivated me. In fact, I'll call her—even if that incurs the wrath of Khan.

My search for platonic male/female friendship will go on—because hope springs eternal. I'm just not going to find it.

Might as well abstain until I'm ready for intimacy once again.

Route 66

Haven't done it, yet. For years I've wanted to drive Route 66. In its entirety—"from Chicago to L.A." (and bring Nat Cole's rendition along for the ride.)
What's the hook here? Let's explore the possibilities. Then we'll draw our conclusions.
Ahhh!! Driving the open road (even without a convertible). Windows down; sunroof open; radio blaring. The smell of gasoline amidst pine trees. Caught the mood?
More often than not, I'm ready to take the long drive. To nowhere in particular. So I might as well have a destination, or scenery along the way.
That's where the "Route 66" dream comes into play. I figure it's one or more of the following:
   a. Wanderlust;
   b. The air-in-the-hair;
   c. Escaping the humdrum;
   d. Experiencing pre-70's Americana;
   e. Donning Ray-Bans and playing James Dean (*Rebel Without a Cause*).
I really like the James Dean thing. (Acting-out again. The dramatic side of me.) With all the affectations. Full-blown individualism.

Since I'm naturally so far-removed from James Dean, it's a chance for me to experience "cool" by learning the role. Wow!! Stopping at a Roswell N.M. greasy-spoon to play billiards, a Winston dangling from the corner of my mouth. No smile—just a smirk.

Of course, little things give me away. Like: persistently curly Jewish hair; wrong rhythm in the walk; deeply-ingrained N.J. accent.

But I'm working on those flaws:
1. Curly Hair (just cut it all off).
2. The "Walk" (Just stand around without moving too much).
3. The "Talk" (Been practicing my Southern drawl—something I picked-up during my days as a prison-riding defense attorney).

So I'm ready-to-roll! Got my plan and got my car.

Has to be my car. Renting one would destroy everything. I can't explain it—except to observe that my car is an extension of my body and my psyche. Not bringing it along is tantamount to depriving it and myself of an inseparable experience.

Back to Earth, Boyer.

"Route 66" is a bit more than just cruising the highway of nostalgia. Beneath the asphalt surface is a REAL America beyond the pre-fab sterility of fast food and ATMs. It's a means of reconnection with people, places, food, and other sensory inputs. A road back to humanity, if you please.

Read this over. Think about it.

Dictionary of Automobiles

I've been chomping-at-the-bit to write this down. It's been in my head for months—and the idea for years.

Cars can be defined. Not by the number of cylinders and horsepower, but by the people who drive them. I'm taking this beyond the guy car/chic car labels into more esoteric categories. Like: professions; dating; ethnicity; and other bullshit.

I mean, you have to know what fits before you buy. The wrong fit will only drive you crazy, and stifle your natural energies. We wouldn't want that, would we?

In order to make this guide user-friendly, I've indexed makes and models under particular traits and applications. There are exceptions due to unusual circumstances. By and large, however, the categories ring true:

I. Heavy Testosterone:
    1. Corvette (not convertible).
    2. Viper (any rendition).
    3. Porsche 911 (Turbo only).
    4. Mustang Cobra w/5-speed. (including Saleen and Steeda packages).

II. Professorial to point of Detachment:
1. Saab 9.3 (without question).
2. Volvo S-60 (base model with cloth).
3. Infiniti I-35. (in white).
4. Oldsmobile Intrigue (any color).

III. I'm Horny (female):
1. Jaguar XK8 (convertible).
2. Porsche Boxster (silver or blue).
3. VW Beetle (yellow).
4. Any Pontiac Firebird (Buy it now. It's the last year).

IV. Cars to me are just Transportation:
1. Dodge Neon (hands-down winner).
2. Mitsubishi Galant.
3. Isuzu Rodeo. (2-wheel drive).
4. Any Saturn.

V. Teen Racers:
1. Honda Civic (w/teeny-tiny wheels).
2. Acura Integra (w/even smaller wheels).
3. Ford Focus (electric blue's the ticket).
4. Any 3-seriers Bimmer.

VI. Senior Rides:

1. Mercury Grand Marquis (with vinyl carriage roof—a must!).
2. Buick Century (aptly named).
3. Toyota Camry (w/cloth).
4. Honda Accord (w/ the black plastic door handles).

Of course, used (sorry—'pre-owned') cars are in a separate category—and relate to other personality traits. The list is exhaustive. Here are a few select picks:

1. Mercedes SL (the sports car): for those who would rather be in the Hamptons or
 Vinyard, but can't afford to get there.
2. Any Used Volvo: typically in hands of computer geek or engineer who believes in things sensible. Can show you why with equations.
3. Original VW Beetle: The King of all time!! Can only belong to a '60s Dropout!!

Well, there you have it, folks. Remember—you saw it here. The first and only "Dictionary of Automobiles." Bet you wish you'd thought of it first!

Superficial though they are, cars have always been a fascinating part of my life; and a constant through the years, changes, and travails.
Very fitting to have that last section cap-off my topics. Yeah—that's it. No more humor left in the 'ole noggin.
You guessed right: time to reflect.

Each Day is a New Day..........Enjoy the Moment

How peaceful it is at 4 in the morning. No phones; no garbage trucks. Just you and the little magnified sounds, reminding us that another day is around the corner. Ready to go—but not just yet.

The sun inevitably rises again. Sadly, its message of hope is obscured by anxiety. Like a persistent/chronic hangover, the aches and pains of daily worries intrude and renew their grip on our lives.

What is "Worry"? How can you and I define it, aside from the textbooks?

I think "worry", fundamentally, is anticipation of future events. Could be something 3 hours or 3 weeks from now; its all the same. Trying to gauge and develop scenarios for coping with consequences not yet apparent. No wonder we're all so fatigued even before our work day begins. We've already depleted the limited reservoirs of energy...on "worry".

The Books tell us too much worry is no good, but a little is healthy. To search for balance. To Hell with that bullshit!

I've never come across anyone who's achieved 'balance'. I say: "Don't worry (at all)! Be Happy!!" (Thank you, Bobby McFerrin.)

Your world won't implode and fall apart. Repeat: *won't fall apart.*

Learn how to Enjoy the Moment. It's been waiting patiently for you all along:

1. People you pass on the sidewalks and streets (smile at them—greet them—converse and listen).
2. Songs on the radio (Listen to the words).
3. The sounds and smells of nature (open your senses).
4. Stories beyond the Headlines (skip the news).
5. (You add to the List).

Begin to experience being alive, not just 'handling' life's problems. Without alcohol or narcotics. Plunge headlong into the process.

To accomplish this, remember—*you have to slow down.*

It's not difficult. Breathe deeply. Fill-up your lungs. I'll bet your chest muscles are constricted. Feel them lose their grip.

You'll need to consciously "restart" every few minutes or so, as old habits hang-on tenaciously. Undoubtedly, this is annoying. But keep the jumper cables ready at all times. Breathing deeply will become second nature—if you give it a real chance.

Now you've set the stage. The rest is up to you. Life's a menu, friend: appetizers, entrees, and desserts. Try one of each, or the full-course meal. Experience what you were meant to be. Just slow down.

Enjoy!!

Epilogue
Aventura, Florida February 27, 2002

I'm finished writing, and haven't had a windfall of cash. That's why this isn't datelined from Main Street, Breckenridge, Colorado. The dream's alive, though, waiting in the wings.

I feel much better. Writing it all down has a certain cathartic effect. Kind of makes some sense out of the jumble.

My daughter (while ever-encouraging me along) says no one wants to read just another "self-help" book—I guess that's what this is. I don't think she's right.

At the supreme risk of sounding immodest, this isn't just another helper-outer. It's supposed to be funny and self-deprecating. I think it's very funny. (*Note: my ex-girlfriend/ex-fiancee once said, emphatically, that I'm *not* funny. She won't be swayed by this book, so I'm not sending her a copy. There!).

If a page or two did indeed make you chuckle, I'm pleased.

Just one small request in return: recommend this book to others. I'm still collecting pennies for the coffee shop.

Bye!!

Printed in the United States
23996LVS00001B/244-270